"Why do I always feel tired, even after a full night's sleep?"

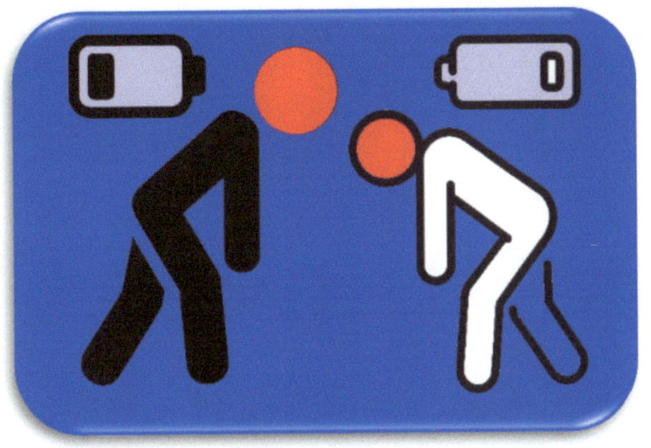

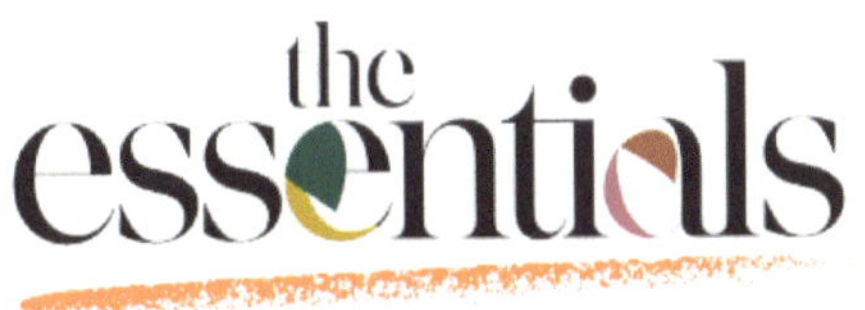

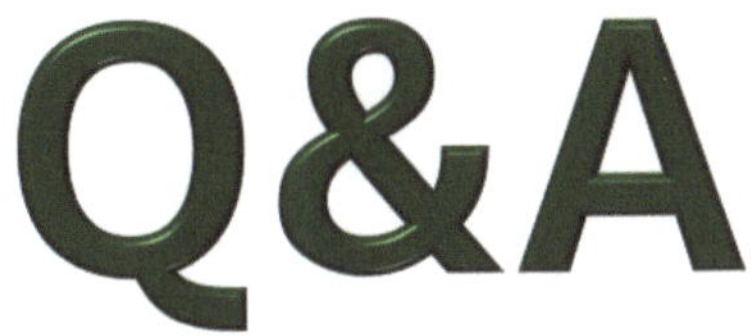

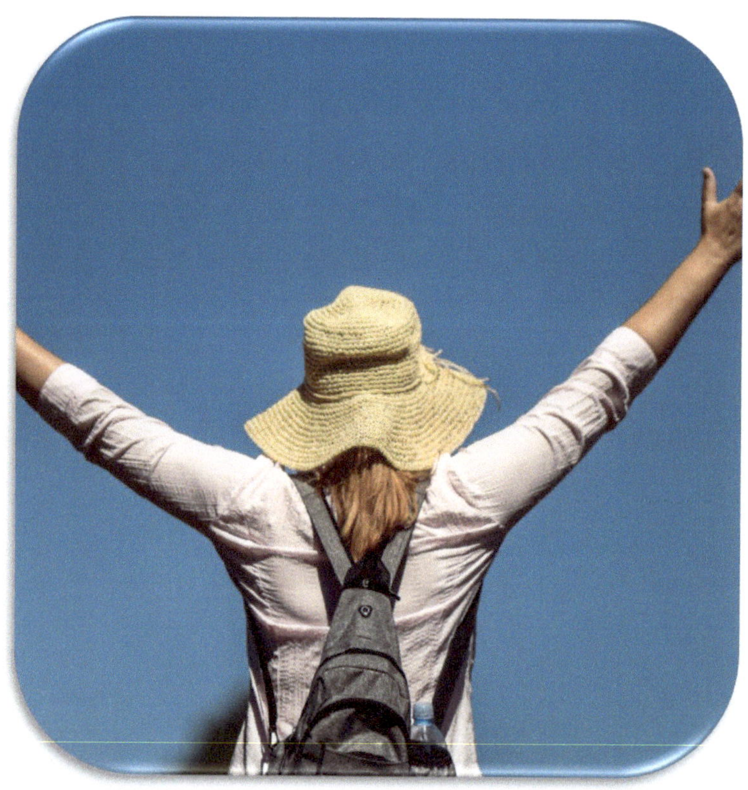

"Our bodies are our gardens; our wills are our gardeners."

William Shakespeare, English playwright, poet & actor

Disclaimer

Please be informed that every effort has been made to ensure the accuracy and completeness of the information presented in this text. However, error is inevitable, and we apologize in advance for any typographical errors or factual inaccuracies that may have inadvertently slipped through. We kindly request that readers bring any such errors to our attention, and we will promptly correct them.

Similarly, when applicable, we have strived to properly attribute all textual and visual content. If any credits have been omitted or misattributed, please inform us so that we may rectify the oversight.

It is important to note that this collection does not purport to be an exhaustive exploration of the subject matter. To delve deeper into specific topics and explore additional resources, we encourage readers to consult the references and further reading suggestions provided.

No commercial agreements were concluded, and no financial incentives, gifts, or compensations were received for the inclusion of any individuals, companies, brands, or services/products. Their presence serves solely the purposes of this book/eBook and does not constitute endorsement or sponsorship.

Foreword

Welcome to this new volume of **the essentials-Q&A**, a series designed to provide clear, concise, and precise answers to the most frequently asked questions of our time, particularly online and on social networks.

Our goal is to provide a concise overview of the current state-of-the-art and to make complex topics accessible to a wide audience, fostering a deeper understanding of the world around us.

the essentials, our new collection, is designed and directed by **Renaud Neurtolz**. Author, editor and technical translator for almost 15 years, Renaud is literally, as his brother-in-law puts it, a "Renaissance man". To date, his writings on a variety of subjects have been sold in 8 countries (Belgium, Canada, France, Germany, Luxembourg, Netherlands, Spain, Switzerland, and the USA).

Curious about everything, passionate about general culture and human creativity in all its forms, as well as the wonders of nature, Renaud is the ideal candidate to manage and develop this collection, whose spirit suits him perfectly. When his "French touch" meets the world and brings it to you through **the essentials**, we can only hope for the best!

the essentials collection is made up of several categories (**the essentials-Essay, the essentials-Knowledge, the essentials-People** and **the essentials-Q&A**) to bring everyone the style of reading they like best.

In addition, recognizing that people learn in different ways, we produce, by ourselves or in collaboration, **videos** and **podcasts** (on our YouTube channel @thessentialscollection), offering alternative perspectives and additional information on the various topics we cover.

The **podcast** and **video** will not be identical to the **eBook** and **printed book** version (available on Amazon) but will be variations of the same subject that will help provide different viewpoints and better memorize the theme thanks to the stimulation of several of our senses (by reading, listening and watching). Moreover, we plan to have them translated into several major languages in the future...

This collection is a testament to our commitment to knowledge dissemination. We believe that everyone, regardless of their background, deserves access to information that is both accurate, informative, and engaging. Through this series, we hope to spark curiosity, inspire critical thinking, and empower individuals to make informed decisions.

As you delve into the different volumes of this collection, you will encounter a diverse range of subjects, from the latest advancements in technology to the timeless wisdom of philosophical thought. Each piece has been carefully crafted to provide a balanced perspective, drawing on the expertise of leading thinkers and researchers.

We invite you to embark on this intellectual and emotional journey with us. May you find the insights within these pages as enlightening as we did when designing them.

We deeply thank you for your trust, time, support, and feedback!

the essentials

A word from the editor...

Believe me, I know what it is like to feel exhausted after a full night's sleep! In the course of researching, designing, and writing this book, I have learned some new and interesting things. I apply some of them in my daily routine (deep breathing, "grounding", exercise, intermittent fasting...) and I must admit that it helps me a lot to improve my energy level and general well-being! I hope you too will find answers and solutions in these pages that will help you live better every day, because each day counts!

Please, feel free to consult the various resources on this subject (eBook, printed book, video, and podcast), which will provide you with a range of interesting perspectives.

Thank you for your confidence and enthusiasm! 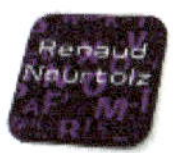

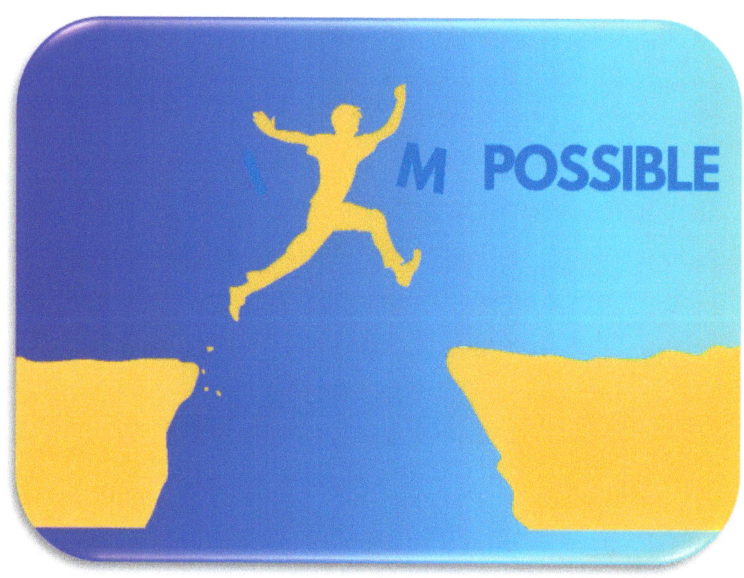

"Nothing is impossible, the word itself says, I'm possible!"

Audrey Hepburn, British actress

Important note

This book is for general knowledge and informational purposes only and does not constitute medical advice. The information provided should not be considered a substitute for professional medical guidance.

Always consult with a qualified healthcare professional for any health concerns or before making any decisions regarding your health or taking any actions after reading some information, particularly taking supplements (that could lead to potential drug interactions, allergies, side effects, etc.) or engaging in specific physical activities (such as high-impact exercises, strenuous workouts, etc.) that could put you at risk, especially if you already have acute or chronic health concerns (pregnancy, any pre-existing medical conditions...).

The publisher, editor and author assume no responsibility for any errors or omissions in this book and disclaim any liability for any injuries or damages resulting from the use of the information contained herein.

Testimonials, examples, and visuals (photos, pictures, diagrams, drawings, etc.) are provided for illustrative purposes only and do not guarantee similar results. Individual results may vary since we are all unique.

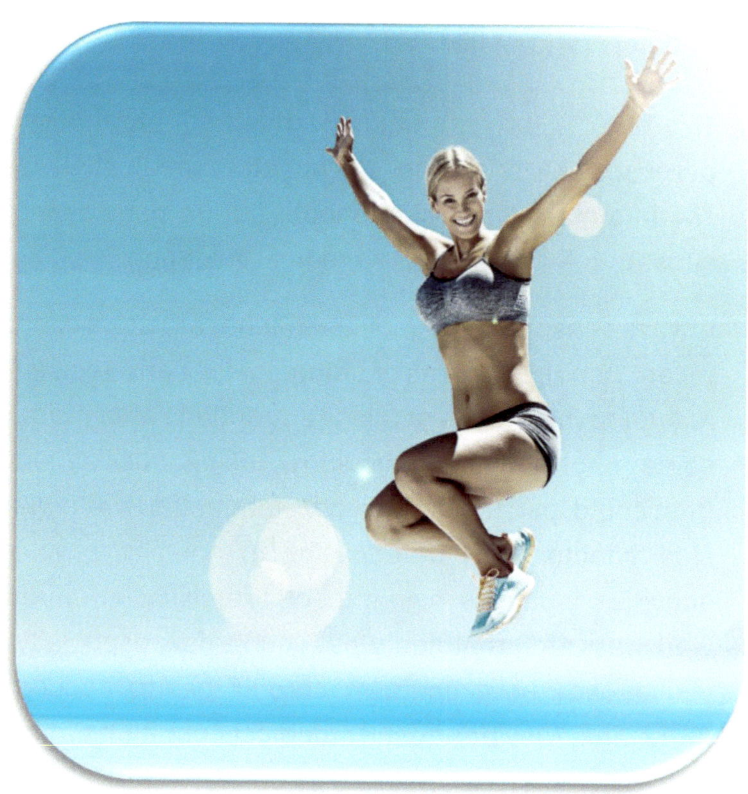

"Wellness is the complete integration of body, mind, and spirit – the realization that everything we do, think, feel, and believe has an effect on our state of well-being."

Greg Anderson, founder & chairman of the Cancer Recovery Foundation

Table of contents

Illustration credits & references

A special thanks for the following online resources that have helped shape the visual world of this document and make its contents so much better!

- ✓ https://www.canva.com
  (Canva Pro version: for some original & altered illustrations)

- ✓ https://notebooklm.google.com
  (Public version: for our "mini podcasts")

- ✓ https://ai.invideo.io
  (Invideo AI Plus: for our short videos)

- ✓ https://gemini.google.com
  (Public version: for some content creation)

- ✓ https://chat.mistral.ai/chat
  (public version: for some content creation)

- ✓ https://chatgpt.com/gpts
  (Public version: for some content creation)

- ✓ https://claude.ai
  (Public version: for some content creation)

Specifically for this printed book, eBook, and PDF:

- ✓ https://www.frontiersin.org/journals/neurology

- ✓ https://www.sleepfoundation.org

- ✓ https://en.wikipedia.org

- ✓ https://wellbeing.gmu.edu

- ✓ https://www.primalhealthcoach.com

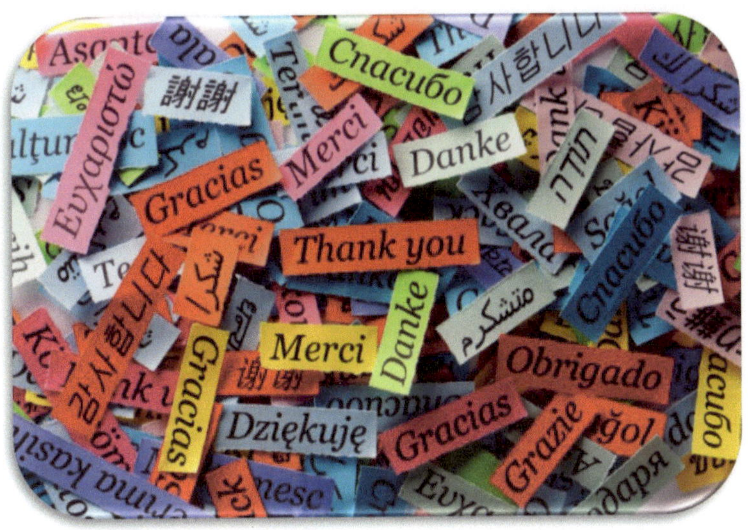

Document information

✓ Title: **"Why do I always feel tired, even after a full night's sleep?"** – V1.0 – the essentials-Q&A – Renaud Neurtolz – December 31, 2024.

✓ ISBN: 9798305360653.

"Take care of your body. It's the only place you have to live."

Emanuel J. Rohn, American entrepreneur, author & motivational speaker

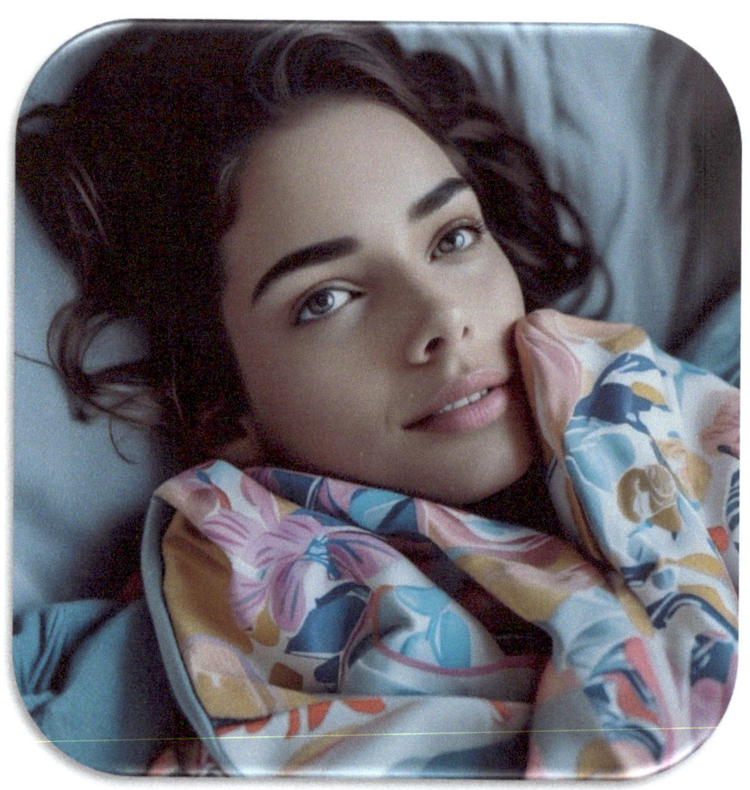

"Having peace, happiness, and healthiness is my definition of beauty. And you can't have any of that without sleep."

Beyoncé, American singer, songwriter & businesswoman

Introduction

Tired of waking up feeling more exhausted than when you went to bed? You are not alone! Feeling persistently tired despite sufficient sleep is a common concern. These "daytime sleepiness" and tiredness can significantly impact quality of life, productivity, and overall well-being.

This new volume of **the essentials-Q&A** explores some of the surprising and often overlooked reasons why you might be chronically fatigued, even after a full night's sleep. We will delve into the latest research on sleep disorders, nutritional deficiencies, hormonal imbalances, medical conditions, lifestyle factors and more that can drain your energy. Get ready to uncover the root of your fatigue and reclaim the vibrant, energized life you deserve.

We hope this reading will equip you with the knowledge and tools to understand your body's unique needs and implement practical and efficient strategies to boost your energy levels and improve your overall well-being!

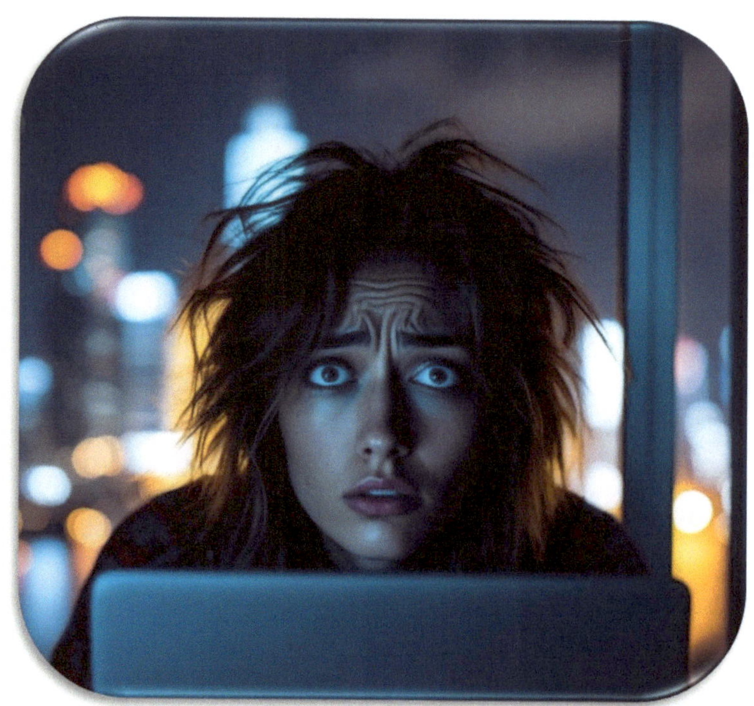

"A sad soul can kill you quicker, far quicker than a germ."

John E. Steinbeck, American writer (Nobel Prize in Literature)

Chapter 1: Common causes of fatigue despite a good night's sleep

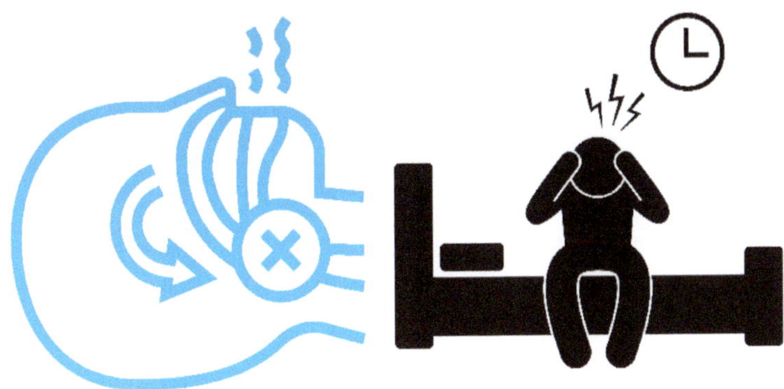

1.1 Sleep disorders

- ✓ **Sleep apnea:** This condition involves pauses in breathing during sleep, disrupting sleep cycles.

  - ○ **Solutions:** Consult a sleep specialist for diagnosis (polysomnography). Treatment options include Continuous Positive Airway Pressure (CPAP) therapy, oral appliances, and in some cases, surgery.

- ✓ **Insomnia:** Difficulty falling asleep, staying asleep, or waking up too early can lead to chronic sleep deprivation.

- ○ **Solutions:**

  - **Cognitive Behavioral Therapy for Insomnia (CBT-I):** A structured program to address negative thoughts and behaviors related to sleep.

  - **Sleep hygiene:** Establish a regular sleep schedule, create a relaxing bedtime routine, optimize your sleep environment (dark, quiet, cool), and avoid screen time before bed.

✓ **Restless Legs Syndrome (RLS):** An overwhelming urge to move the legs, often accompanied by uncomfortable sensations.

- ○ **Solutions:** Medications, lifestyle adjustments (regular exercise, warm baths), and iron supplementation (if iron deficiency is present).

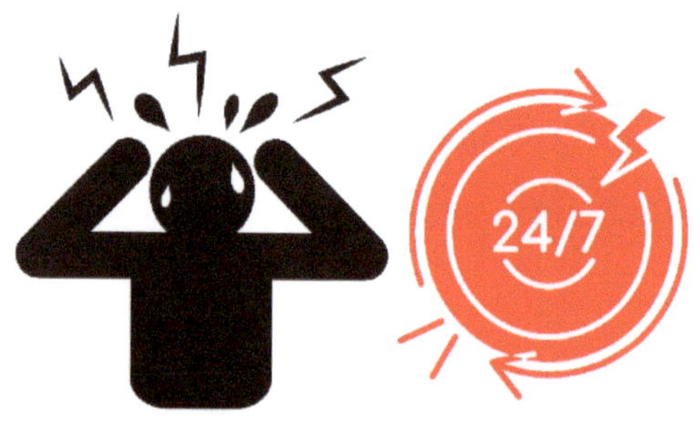

1.2 Medical conditions

- ✓ **Hypothyroidism:** An underactive thyroid gland can cause fatigue, weight gain, and slow metabolism.

- ✓ **Anemia:** Iron deficiency can lead to fatigue due to insufficient oxygen delivery to tissues (iron deficiency anemia).

- ✓ **Chronic Fatigue Syndrome (CFS):** A complex disorder characterized by persistent fatigue that is not improved by rest.

- ✓ **Depression/anxiety:** Fatigue is a common symptom of depression, often accompanied by low mood, loss of interest, and difficulty concentrating.

- ✓ **Diabetes:** Uncontrolled blood sugar levels can cause fatigue, especially in people with type 1 or type 2 diabetes.

- ✓ **Heart conditions:** Certain heart problems, such as congestive heart failure, can lead to fatigue due to reduced blood flow to the body.

- ✓ **Vitamin D deficiency:** Can increase the risk of sleep disorders and is associated with sleep difficulties, shorter sleep duration, nocturnal awakenings, fatigue, and depression.

✓ **Magnesium deficiency:** Higher levels of magnesium in the body are associated with better sleep, longer sleep times, and less tiredness during the day. Studies of older adults also found that magnesium supplementation helped with falling asleep faster and protected against waking up earlier than intended.

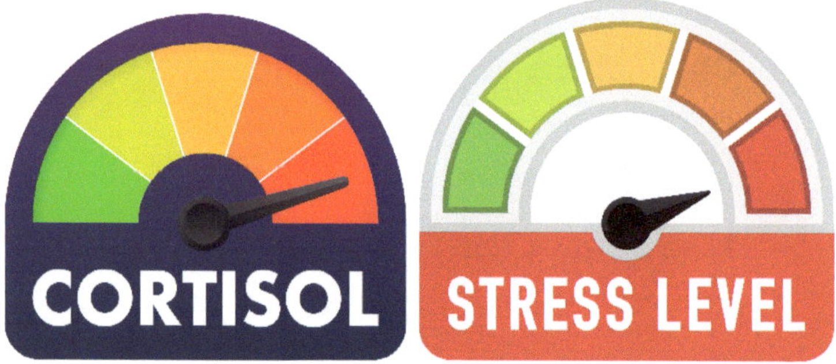

1.3 Lifestyle factors

✓ **Poor diet:** A diet lacking in essential nutrients (iron, vitamin B12, vitamin D, magnesium) can contribute to fatigue.

○ **Solutions:** Focus on whole foods, including fruits, vegetables, lean protein, and whole grains. Consider supplements under the guidance of a healthcare professional.

- ✓ **Lack of exercise/sedentary behavior (or overtraining!):** Regular physical activity can improve sleep quality and increase energy levels.

  - ○ **Solutions:** Aim for at least 150 minutes of moderate-intensity or 75 minutes of vigorous-intensity aerobic activity per week.

- ✓ **Dehydration:** Dehydration can lead to fatigue, dizziness, and decreased cognitive function.

  - ○ **Solutions:** Drink water containing sufficient minerals/electrolytes, in the right proportions.

- ✓ **Excessive stress/mental load:** Chronic stress, work stress, family responsibilities, financial worries, etc., can disrupt sleep and contribute to fatigue (linked to high levels of cortisol, the stress hormone that can interfere with sleep and well-being when elevated).

  - ○ **Solutions:** Practice stress-reduction techniques such as mindfulness meditation, deep breathing exercises, yoga, spending time in nature, etc.

- ✓ **Substance abuse:** Alcohol consumption and drug use can significantly disrupt sleep patterns.

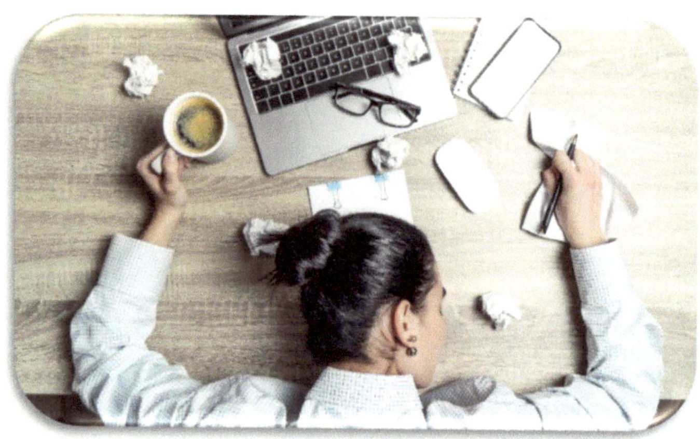

1.4 Other factors

- ✓ **Age:** Fatigue is more common in older adults due to changes in sleep patterns and hormonal imbalances.

- ✓ **Medications:** Some medications can cause fatigue as a side effect.

- ✓ **Shift work:** Working night shifts can disrupt the body's natural circadian rhythm, leading to sleep disturbances and fatigue.

- ✓ **Environmental factors**: Temperature, noise, (artificial) light pollution, seasonal changes, poor air quality, electromagnetic pollution...

- ✓ **Information overload:** Occurs when the brain exceeds its capacity to process information. This can make you feel tired and overwhelmed.

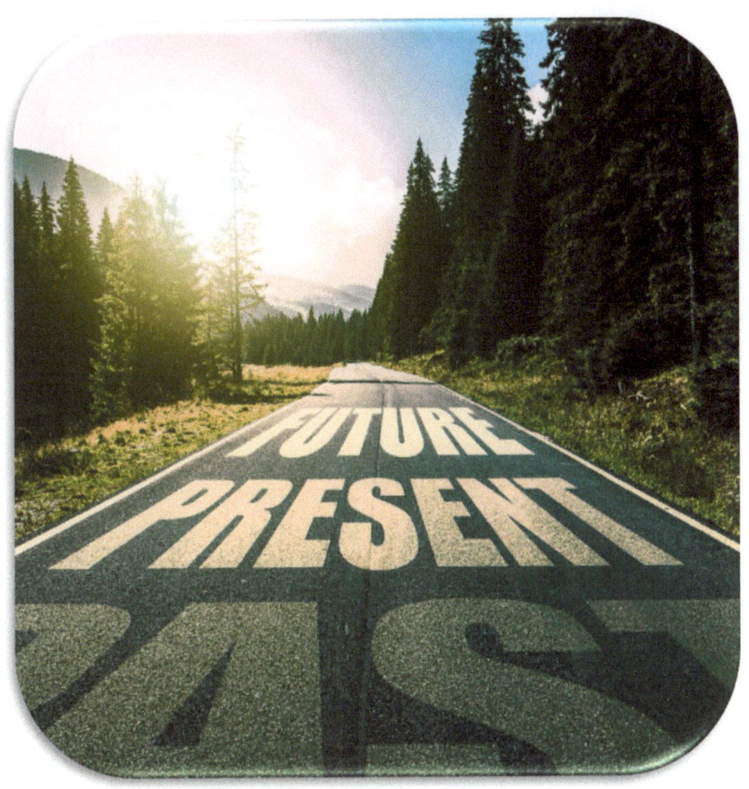

"Don't let the past steal your present."

Cherríe Moraga, American Chicana feminist, writer, activist, poet

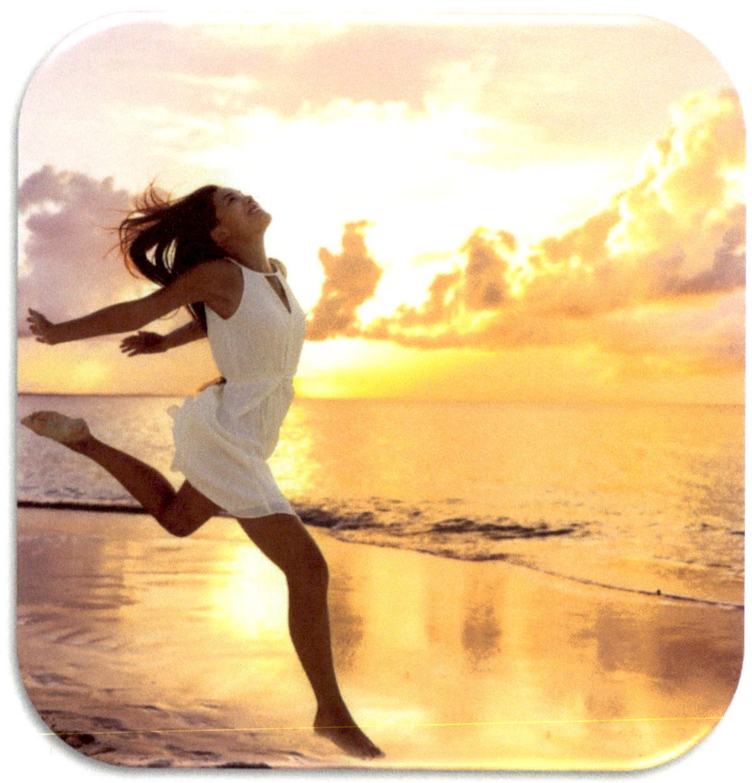

"A well spent day brings happy sleep."

Leonardo di ser Piero da Vinci, Italian polymath of the Renaissance

Chapter 2: Solutions & interventions

Optimal Sleep Environment

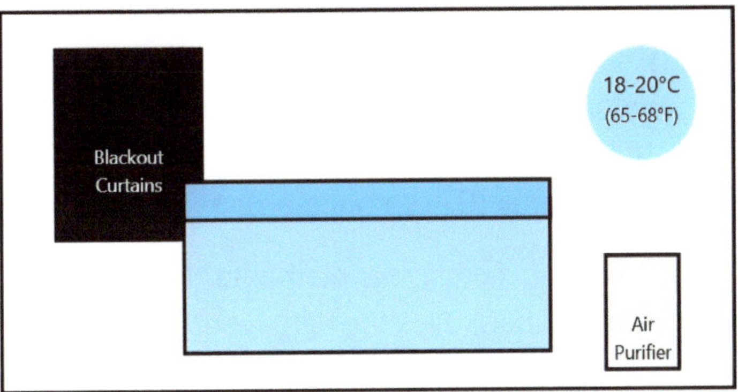

2.1 Immediate actions

2.1.1 Sleep optimization

- ✓ Maintain consistent sleep/wake times.

- ✓ Create a dark and cool sleeping environment (18-20°C) with fresh air.

- ✓ Practice a wind-down routine.

- ✓ Invest in quality mattress and pillows.

2.1.2 Nutrition essentials

- ✓ Stay well hydrated (water with enough minerals).

✓ Eat balanced meals with high-quality proteins, complex carbs, healthy fats, and fiber.

✓ Do not eat 3 to 4 hours before going to bed.

✓ If your health permits, try intermittent fasting. Surprisingly and counter-intuitively, it can give you more energy, reduce fatigue, increase mental sharpness, well-being (while helping control your weight….), etc. Consult your general practitioner (GP) before starting.

✓ Consider taking supplements (after medical consultation). Pick the right type/form for you:

   o Vitamin D3 (with K2).

   o B-complex vitamins.

   o Magnesium (citrate, gluconate, etc.).

   o Iron (if proven deficiency).

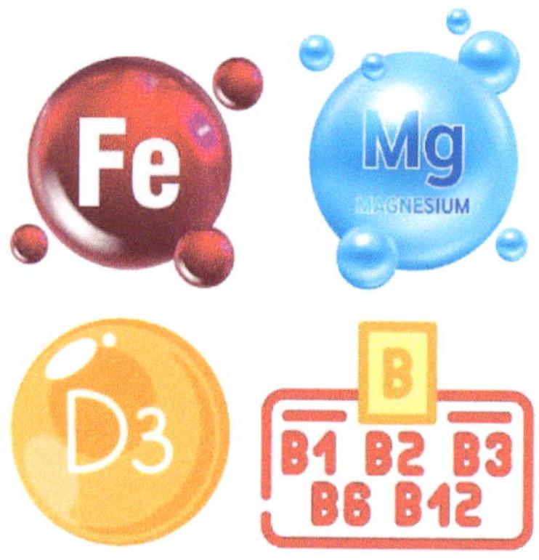

2.2 Lifestyle changes

2.2.1 Movement and exercise

- ✓ Regular moderate exercise (150 minutes/week).
- ✓ Daily walk (minimum 30 minutes).
- ✓ Regular stretching.
- ✓ Avoid sitting for long periods.

2.2.2 Stress management

- ✓ Daily meditation (10-20 minutes).
- ✓ Deep breathing exercises.
- ✓ Regular breaks during work.
- ✓ Nature exposure ("grounding").

2.2.3 Digital wellness

- ✓ Screen-free time before bed.
- ✓ Regular digital detox periods.
- ✓ Blue light filtering.

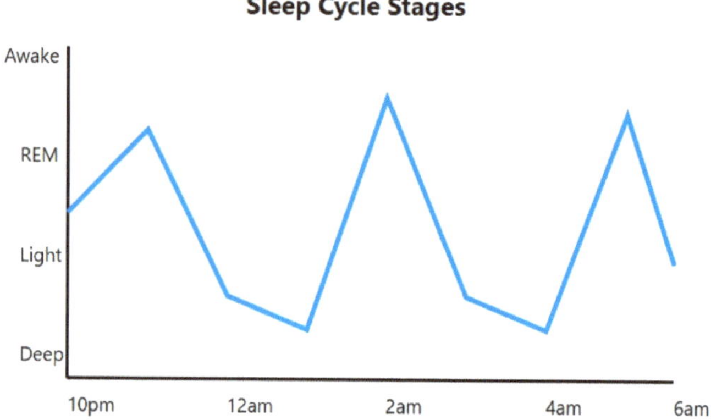

2.3 Quick energy boosters and well-being tips

- ✓ **Optimize your sleep environment:** Make sure your bedroom is dark, quiet, cool and has clean air.

- ✓ **Establish a regular sleep schedule:** Go to bed and wake up at the same time each day, even on weekends.

- ✓ **Create a relaxing bedtime routine:** Take a warm bath, read a book, or listen to calming music before bed.

- ✓ **Avoid caffeine and alcohol before bed.**

- ✓ **Limit screen time before bed.**

- ✓ **Get regular exercise.**

✓ **Eat a healthy diet.**

✓ **Stay hydrated** (get enough minerals).

✓ **Practice stress-reduction techniques** (yoga, meditation, relaxation, self-hypnosis).

✓ **Consider natural remedies:** Some herbal supplements, such as valerian root and chamomile, may promote relaxation and improve sleep quality.

Optimal Daily Energy Schedule

Morning Routine 6-9 AM Hydrate, Exercise, Sunlight	Peak Performance 9-1 PM Important Tasks, Meetings	Afternoon Reset 1-5 PM Light Tasks, Breaks	Evening Routine 5-9 PM Wind Down, Relaxation

2.4 Morning routine

2.4.1 First 30 minutes

✓ Drink 2 glasses of water (approx. 400/500 ml) with a pinch of quality sea salt or Himalayan pink salt or any other quality salt/mineral blend that provides you with all the minerals/electrolytes your body has lost overnight and needs in the morning.

✓ If conditions allow expose yourself to natural sunlight immediately upon waking for 5/10 minutes.

- ✓ Practice 5/10 minutes of deep breathing (3 sets of 30 deep breaths with a pause on the exhalation and inhalation until you can't hold it anymore between each series). Ideally outdoor or in a room with fresh clean air (opened window if you have a garden/park around).

- ✓ If conditions allow walk/stand barefoot on natural grass (or earth) for a few minutes (you can do it with your deep breathing exercises and sun exposure). This practice is known as "grounding" or "earthing".

- ✓ Practice 5 minutes of light stretching.

- ✓ Avoid checking phone/emails until after breakfast (or after your morning routine if you skip breakfast/practice intermittent fasting).

2.4.2 Nutrition kickstart

- ✓ Eat protein-rich breakfast within 1 hour of waking (for those eating breakfast/not doing intermittent fasting. Otherwise, it can be during your brunch/lunch).

- ✓ Include healthy fats (avocado, nuts, eggs).

- ✓ Add fermented foods for gut health.

- ✓ Consider morning green tea instead of coffee.

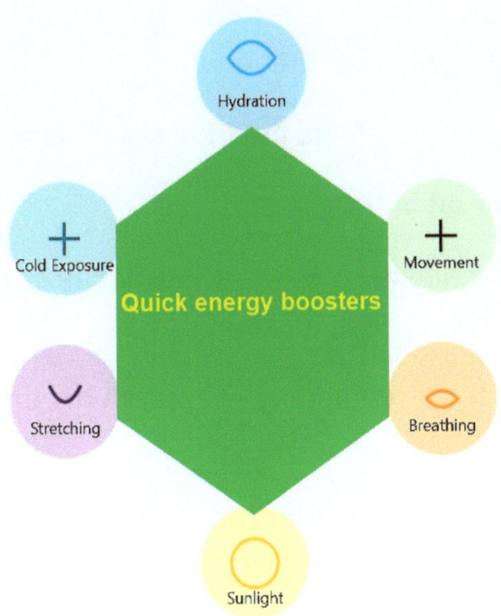

2.5 Throughout the day

2.5.1 Energy management

- ✓ Work in 90-minute focused blocks.

- ✓ Take 10-minute breaks every hour.

- ✓ Stand or walk during phone calls.

- ✓ Use the "2-minute rule": If a task takes less than 2 minutes, do it now.

2.5.2 Physical boosters

- ✓ Cold shower or face splashing.

- ✓ Power posing for 2 minutes.

✓ Quick desk exercises (neck rolls, shoulder shrugs, ankle rotations).

✓ Alternate nostril breathing for 5 minutes.

2.5.3. Mental clarity

✓ Practice the 5-5-5 method: Focus on 5 things you can see, hear, and feel.

✓ Use aromatherapy (peppermint, citrus, cineol rosemary...).

✓ Listen to binaural beats during work or before sleeping (many on YouTube, see the "Resources" section).

✓ Take micro-nature breaks (even looking at plants helps).

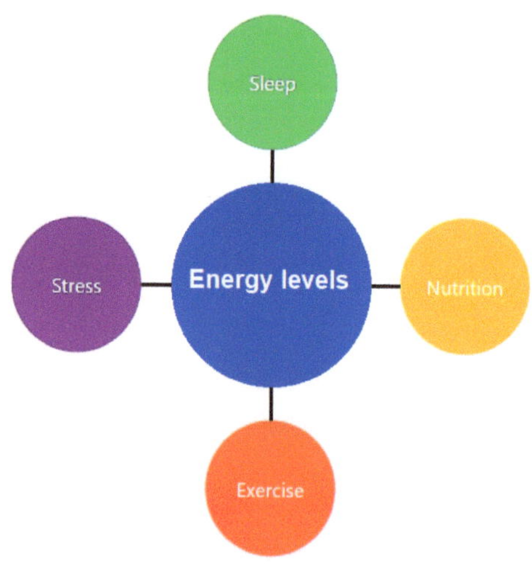

2.6 Evening optimization

2.6.1 Wind-down routine

- ✓ Create a "sunset dimming" routine in your home.

- ✓ Practice progressive muscle relaxation

- ✓ Use magnesium oil spray or bath.

- ✓ Journal three "gratitudes" and "tomorrow's" priorities.

"Sleep is the golden chain that ties health and our bodies together."

Thomas Dekker, English Elizabethan dramatist, pamphleteer & writer

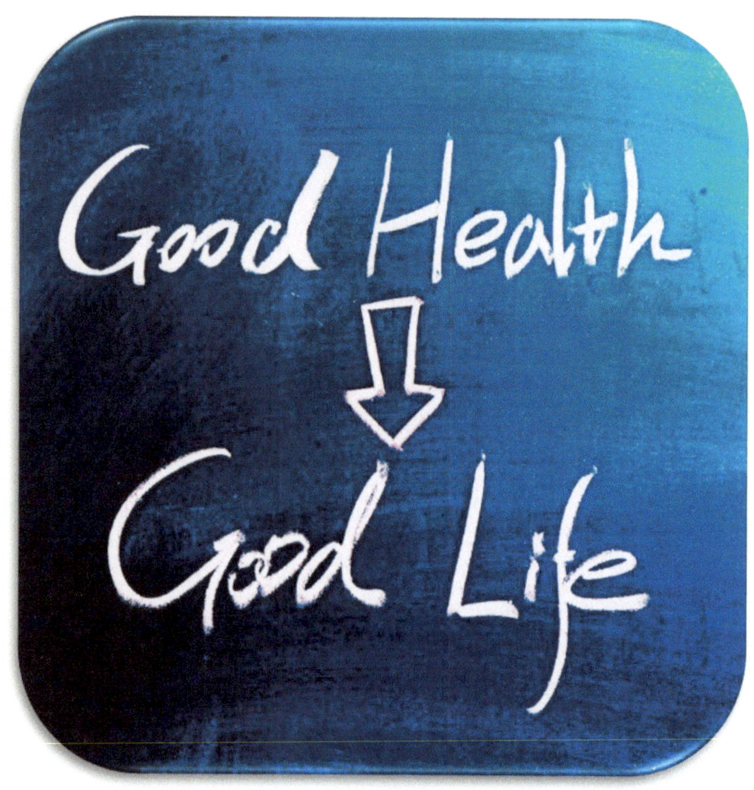

"A year from now, you will wish you had started today."

Karen Lamb, Australian teacher & author

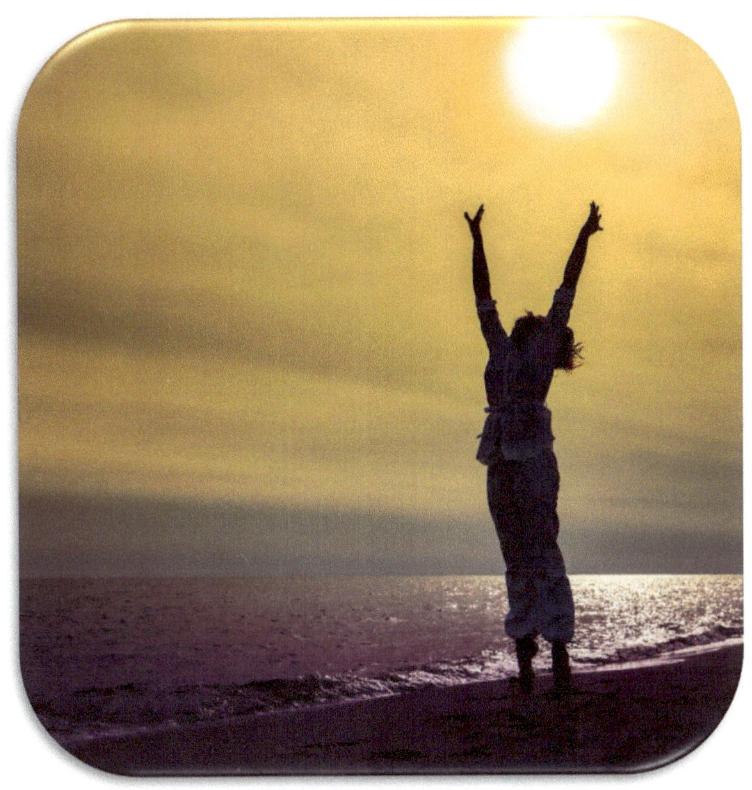

"A calm mind brings inner strength and self-confidence, so that's very important for good health."

Dalai Lama (Tenzin Gyatso), 14th leader of the Tibetan Buddhism

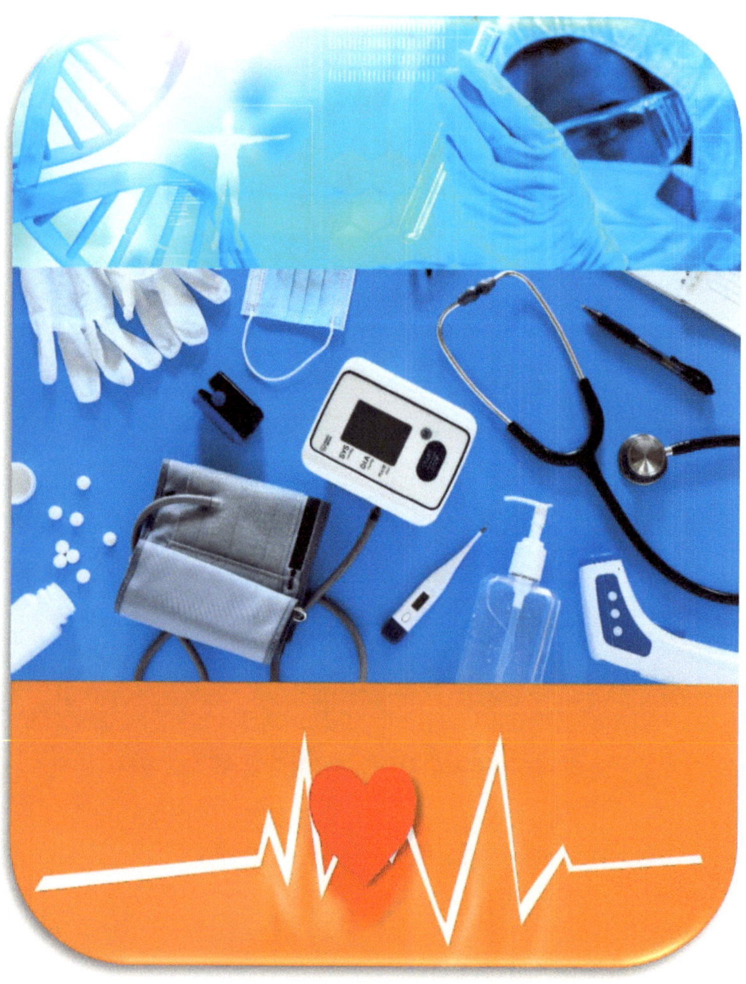

"In order to change we must be sick and tired of being sick and tired."

Anonymous/unknown author

Chapter 3: When to seek professional help?

✓ Persistent fatigue lasting more than 2 weeks.

✓ Accompanying symptoms (unexplained weight changes, repeated pain, inflammation, swelling of any part of the body, excessive sweating, or sudden sensation of intense heat or cold...).

✓ Mental health concerns (such as mood swings, panic attacks, persistent state of depression or chronic stress....).

✓ Persistent sleep disorders symptoms.

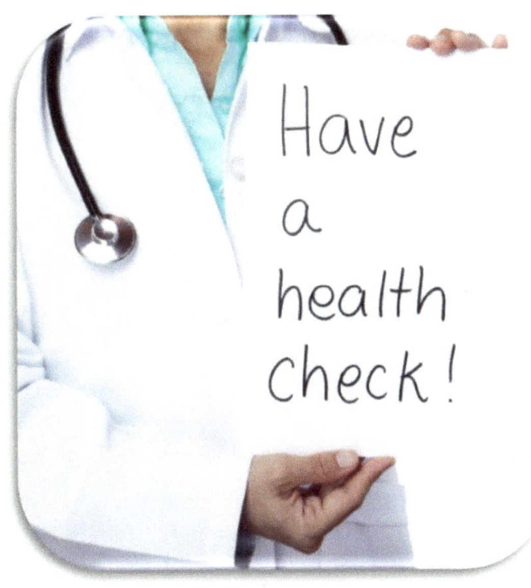

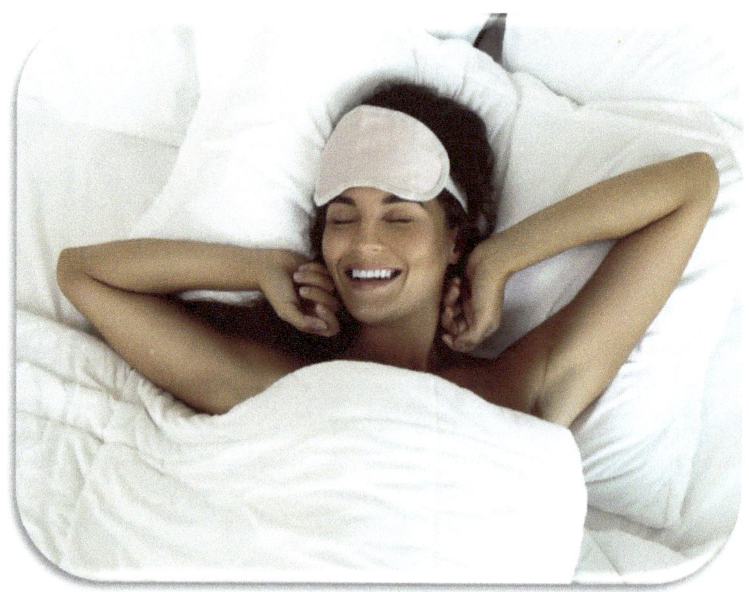

"The best bridge between despair and hope is a good night's sleep."

Eli J. Cossman, American inventor, businessman & author

Resources

- ✓ **Books/eBooks:**

    - ○ "Why We Sleep" by Matthew Walker

    - ○ "The Sleep Solution" by W. Chris Winter

    - ○ "The Power of When" by Michael Breus

    - ○ "The Energy Plan" by James Collins

    - ○ "The Circadian Code" by Satchin Panda

- ✓ **Podcasts:**

    - ○ "Sleep With Me"

    - ○ "The Huberman Lab"

    - ○ "Found My Fitness"

- ✓ **Apps:**

    - ○ **Calm**: Guided meditations and sleep stories: Google Play (Android), App Store (iPhone)

    - ○ **Headspace**: Mindfulness and meditation exercises: Google Play (Android), App Store (iPhone)

- o **Sleep Cycle**: Tracks your sleep patterns and provides personalized insights: Google Play (Android), App Store (iPhone)

- o **MyFitnessPal**: Nutrition tracking: Google Play (Android), App Store (iPhone)

✓ **Documentaries:**

- o "The Truth about of Sleep" (BBC)

- o "The Science of Sleep" (National Geographic)

- o "Take a Deep Breath" (BBC)

✓ **Audio**

- o Binaural beats selection on YouTube (for work, sleep, relaxation…)

"Movement is a medicine for creating change in a person's physical, emotional, and mental states."

Caroline Myss, American author about mysticism & wellness

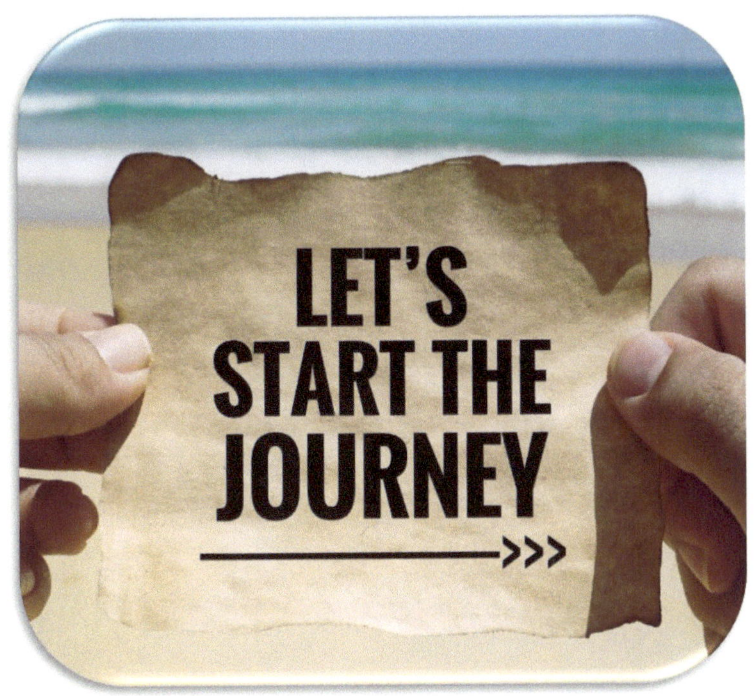

"You can't put a limit on how much you can improve and how much you can do. There are no limits on what you can be, or what you can do, except the limits you place on yourself."

Brian Tracy, Canadian American motivational public speaker & author

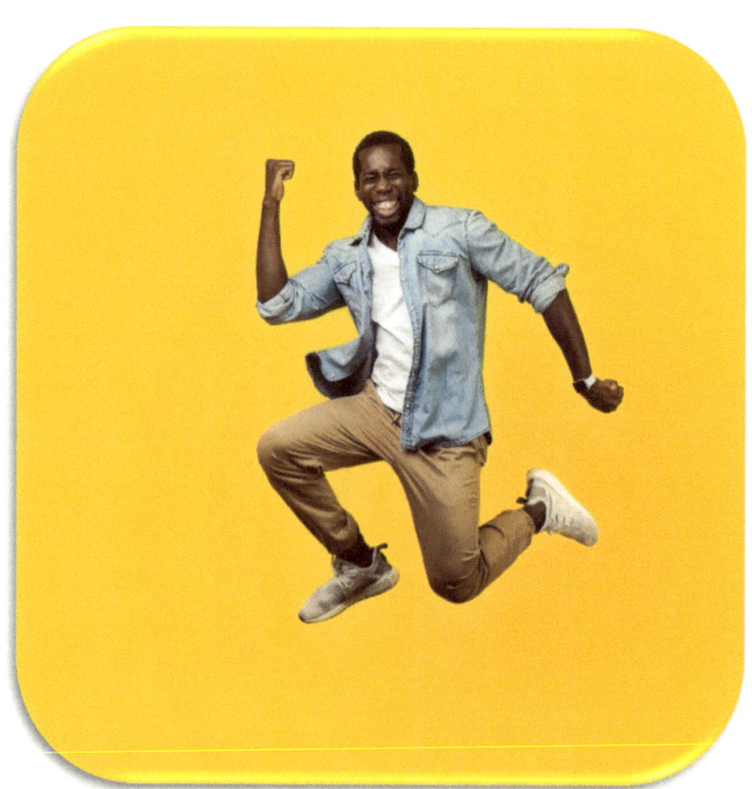

"Those who do not find time for exercise will have to find time for illness."

Earl of Derby

Glossary

A

- ✓ **Adenosine:** A neurochemical that builds up during waking hours, creating sleep pressure.

C

- ✓ **Circadian rhythm:** The natural 24-hour cycle that regulates sleep-wake cycles.

- ✓ **Cognitive Behavioral Therapy for Insomnia (CBT-I):** A type of psychotherapy that helps individuals identify and change negative thoughts and behaviors that interfere with sleep.

- ✓ **Continuous Positive Airway Pressure (CPAP):** A treatment for sleep apnea that uses a machine to deliver pressurized air through a mask, keeping the airway open during sleep.

- ✓ **Cortisol:** Stress hormone that can interfere with sleep when elevated.

D

- ✓ **Dehydration:** A state in which the body loses more fluids than it takes in (also linked to minerals/electrolytes imbalances).

H

- ✓ **Hormones:** Chemical messengers produced by the endocrine glands that regulate various bodily functions.

I

- ✓ **Insomnia:** Difficulty falling asleep, staying asleep, or waking up too early.

M

- ✓ **Melatonin:** Sleep hormone produced in response to darkness.

- ✓ **Metabolism:** The chemical processes that occur within a living organism to maintain life.

- ✓ **Mindfulness:** Paying attention to the present moment without judgment.

P

- ✓ **Polysomnography:** A sleep study that records various physiological activities during sleep, including brain waves, breathing, and heart rate.

R

- ✓ **REM sleep:** Rapid Eye Movement sleep phase crucial for mental restoration.

S

- ✓ **Sleep apnea:** A sleep disorder/condition characterized by repeated pauses in breathing during sleep.

- ✓ **Sleep hygiene:** Practices and habits that promote good sleep quality.

- ✓ **Sleep inertia:** Grogginess and disorientation that can occur after waking.

- ✓ **Slow-wave sleep:** Deep sleep phase essential for physical restoration.

- ✓ **Stress:** A state of mental or emotional strain or tension resulting from adverse or demanding circumstances.

Z

- ✓ **Zeitgeber:** External cue/factor that helps regulate circadian rhythms (e.g., sunlight).

"Let thy food be thy medicine and thy medicine be thy food."

Hippocrates, Greek physician & philosopher of the classical period

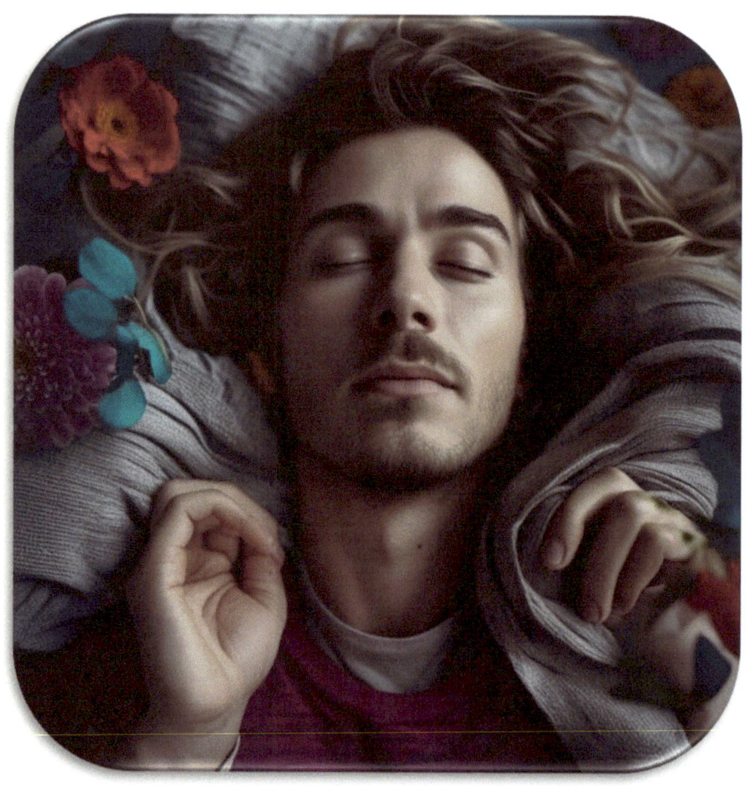

"Health is a state of body. Wellness is a state of being."

Jane E. Stanford, American philanthropist & co-founder of Stanford university

To keep the story going...

The journey to reclaiming your energy may not always be linear, but it's a journey worth taking.

By understanding the root causes of your fatigue and implementing the strategies outlined here, you can begin to break free from the cycle of exhaustion.

Remember to be patient with yourself, celebrate small victories, and prioritize self-care.

You deserve to feel vibrant and energized. This is your starting point – a path towards a healthier, more fulfilling life...

"The higher your energy level, the more efficient your body. The more efficient your body, the better you feel and the more you will use your talent to produce outstanding results."

Tony Robbins, American author, coach & motivational speaker

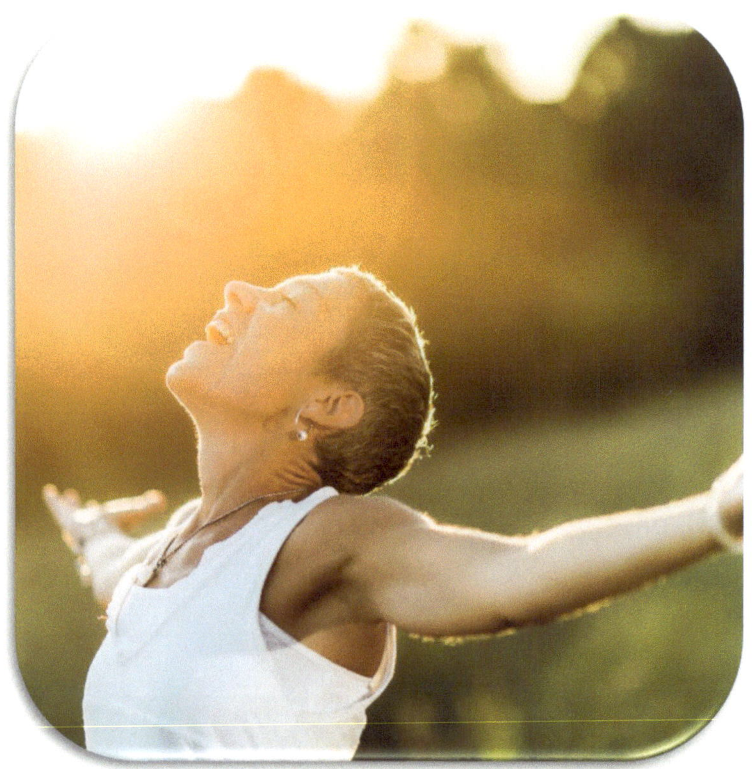

"Physical fitness is not only one of the most important keys to a healthy body; it is the basis of dynamic and creative intellectual activity."

John F. Kennedy, 35th president of the United States

We hope you enjoyed this reading...
Stay tuned for our next exciting topic!!

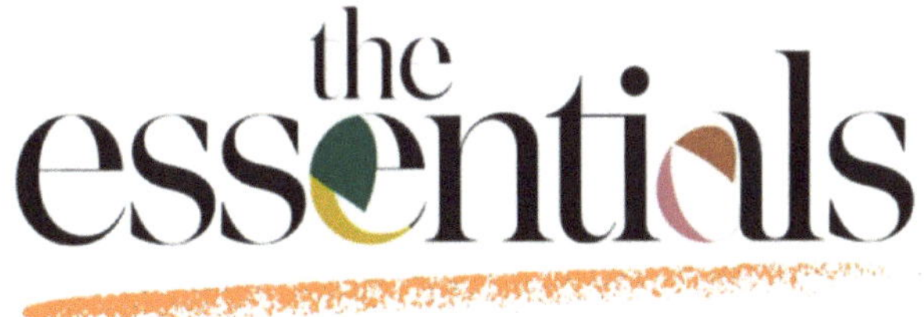

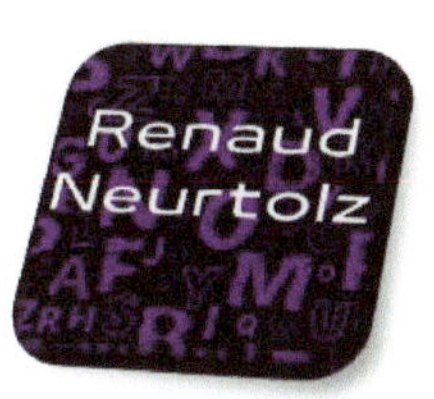